EVERYTHING ABOUT HEPARIN-INDUCED THROMBOCYTOPENIA (HIT)

A Complete Guide For Patients, Caregivers, And Healthcare Professionals - Causes, Symptoms, Diagnosis, Treatment, Coping Strategies, And More

DR. CADE JOSUE

Table of Contents

DISCLAIMER

The information provided in this book is for general informational purposes only. It is not intended as medical advice, diagnosis, or treatment.

The content of this book should not be considered a substitute for professional medical advice. Readers should consult with a qualified healthcare provider for diagnosis and treatment of any medical conditions they have.

While every effort has been made to ensure the accuracy and completeness of the information presented, the author makes no representations or warranties of any kind, express or implied, about the completeness, accuracy, reliability, suitability, or availability with respect to the information, contained in this book.

The author disclaims any responsibility for any loss or damage resulting from reliance on the information provided in this book. References to individuals, products, websites, organizations, or other names are for informational purposes only and do not imply endorsement.

By reading this book, readers acknowledge that they are responsible for their own health decisions and should seek appropriate medical advice when necessary.

ABOUT THIS BOOK

"Everything About Heparin-Induced Thrombocytopenia (HIT)" is an all-encompassing manual that provides invaluable insights into the comprehension and control of this urgent medical condition. Its significance is rooted in the fact that it furnishes students, healthcare professionals, and researchers with a comprehensive and current resource encompassing a multitude of facets associated with HIT.

The introductory chapter of this book, titled "Introduction to Heparin-Induced Thrombocytopenia (HIT)," provides an overview of the subject matter and emphasizes the importance of HIT in the context of clinical practice. By doing so, readers acquire a fundamental comprehension of HIT before exploring more specialized subjects.

An essential subject addressed is "Comprehending Thrombocytopenia and Its Causes," which provides a comprehensive analysis of the pathogenesis underlying low platelet counts and the various etiologies that may contribute to thrombocytopenia, including HIT.

This books "History and Discovery of Heparin-Induced Thrombocytopenia" presents a historical context that elucidates the progressive development of knowledge regarding HIT and its influence on contemporary approaches to diagnosis and management.

This book further explores the categorization of HIT under the heading "Types of Heparin-Induced Thrombocytopenia," offering a comprehensive understanding of the varied clinical manifestations and heterogeneity of this condition.

It is imperative to comprehend the "Mechanisms of HIT Development" to gain insight into the fundamental processes that propel this immune-mediated response, thereby facilitating the development of targeted therapeutic strategies.

Clinical practitioners derive substantial value from the comprehensive examination of "Diagnosis and Laboratory Testing for HIT" and "Clinical Manifestations of HIT," as these sections provide pragmatic recommendations for the identification and validation of HIT within clinical environments.

In "Differential Diagnosis of HIT," this book additionally tackles the complexities associated with differential diagnosis. This section assists healthcare practitioners in differentiating HIT from alternative conditions that exhibit comparable symptoms.

A comprehensive analysis of "Risk Factors for Developing HIT" and "Complications Associated with HIT" provides readers with the necessary information to conduct risk assessments and implement proactive management strategies.

This books "Management and Treatment Strategies for HIT" and "Pharmacological Interventions for HIT" provide in-depth analyses of evidence-based methods, such as innovative therapies and anticoagulant alternatives, which empower readers to maximize the quality of patient care.

This book "Non-pharmacological Approaches for HIT Management" provides insights into supplementary strategies that can enhance the efficacy of pharmacotherapy.

The critical aspects of prognosis and long-term outcomes are addressed in "Prognosis and Long-term Outcomes of HIT," which assists clinicians in comprehending the course of HIT and its effects on the health of patients.

In "Patient Education and Support for HIT" and "Prevention Strategies and Guidelines for HIT," this book further underscores the importance of patient education, support, and preventive measures. This promotes the implementation of holistic care and proactive risk mitigation.

In conclusion, "Everything About Heparin-Induced Thrombocytopenia (HIT)" emerges as an indispensable resource that not only deepens understanding but also informs clinical practice, research endeavors, and patient-centered care in the domain of HIT management.

CHAPTER ONE

Heparin-Induced Thrombocytopenia (HIT): An Introduction

A serious immune-mediated complication of heparin therapy (HIT) is associated with the commonly used anticoagulant heparin. A paradoxical decrease in platelet count and an elevated risk of thrombosis characterize this condition, which can result in arterial thrombosis, pulmonary embolism (PE), deep vein thrombosis (DVT), and deep vein thrombosis (DVT). All of these complications are potentially fatal. HIT typically develops between 5 and 10 days following the commencement of heparin therapy; however, precedent heparin exposure may result in an earlier onset.

There are two distinct classifications for HIT: type I and type II. Typically benign, Type I HIT is a moderate thrombocytopenia that does not involve the immune system and develops within the initial few days following heparin exposure. Conversely, type II HIT is an immune-mediated response characterized by platelet activation and consumption due to the formation of antibodies against heparin-bound platelet factor 4 (PF4). This leads to a substantial reduction in platelet count and an elevated susceptibility to thrombosis.

Clinical suspicion, platelet count monitoring, and laboratory tests for the detection of HIT antibodies are utilized to establish the diagnosis of HIT. It is critical to promptly identify and treat HIT to prevent thrombotic complications. To prevent further thrombosis, treatment consists of discontinuing heparin and initiating alternative anticoagulation therapy, such as direct thrombin inhibitors like fondaparinux or argatroban.

An Overview Of Thrombocytopenia And Its Origins

A thrombocytopenic disorder is distinguished by an extremely diminished platelet count within the bloodstream. Platelets, which are also referred to as thrombocytes, are bone marrow-produced microscopic cell fragments that are essential for hemostasis and blood coagulation. A multitude of underlying factors can contribute to thrombocytopenia, such as heightened sequestration, diminished production, or increased degradation of platelets.

The Following Are Frequent Etiologies Of Thrombocytopenia

1. Platelet production can be impaired in the bone marrow due to conditions such as chemotherapy, certain medications (e.g., alcohol, certain

antibiotics), and bone marrow disorders (e.g., aplastic anemia, leukemia).

2. Platelet destruction induced by the immune system can be heightened in instances like immune thrombocytopenic purpura (ITP), in which platelets are erroneously targeted and eradicated by the immune system. Infections (e.g., hepatitis, HIV), specific medications (e.g., heparin-induced thrombocytopenia), and autoimmune disorders are additional factors that contribute to increased platelet destruction.

3. Elevated sequestration: The spleen may occasionally sequester an abnormally high quantity of platelets, resulting in a reduction of the circulating platelet count. This may transpire in instances of liver cirrhosis, wherein obstruction of the spleen is induced by portal hypertension.

Symptoms of thrombocytopenia may include petechiae (tiny red or purple patches on the skin), easy bruising, mucosal bleeding (nosebleeds, bleeding gums), and, in extreme instances, spontaneous bleeding or hemorrhage. To ascertain the underlying cause of thrombocytopenia, a comprehensive medical history, physical examination, complete blood count (CBC) with peripheral blood smear, and additional laboratory tests are required for diagnosis.

The Origins And Exploration Of Heparin-Mediated Thrombocytopenia

Heparin-induced thrombocytopenia (HIT) originated with the discovery of heparin as an anticoagulant in the early 20th century. Heparin, a glycosaminoglycan with a high degree of sulfation, was first extracted from animal tissues before being synthesized for therapeutic purposes. The anticoagulant properties of the substance were initially identified by William Henry Howell and Jay McLean during the 1920s. They established its capacity to inhibit blood clot formation in vivo and extend coagulation times in vitro.

In the 1950s and 1960s, clinicians observed a paradoxical decline in platelet count among patients undergoing heparin therapy; these were the earliest documented cases of HIT. The immune-mediated mechanism that underlies HIT was not, nevertheless, elucidated until the 1970s. It was found that heparin could stimulate the production of antibodies targeting platelet factor 4 (PF4), a protein that is secreted by platelets that have been activated.

In 1973, C.G. Kelton et al. contributed additional knowledge regarding the pathophysiology of HIT through their demonstration that the presence of heparin-PF4 complexes induced platelet activation and aggregation in response to HIT antibodies. Platelet depletion, thrombocytopenia, and an elevated susceptibility to thrombosis ensued as a consequence. The significance of the

Fc segment of HIT antibodies in facilitating platelet activation through FcγRIIa receptors located on platelet surfaces was established by subsequent research.

Improvements in laboratory testing, including enzyme-linked immunosorbent assays (ELISA) and functional assays, have contributed to the ongoing enhancement of HIT diagnosis. Furthermore, the advancement of alternative anticoagulants, including factor Xa inhibitors (e.g., fondaparinux) and direct thrombin inhibitors (e.g., argatroban, bivalirudin), has significantly transformed the approach to managing HIT. These agents offer efficacious anticoagulation without the potential to worsen thrombocytopenia.

In summary, the discovery and understanding of heparin-induced thrombocytopenia have evolved over several decades, shaping the diagnosis, management, and prevention of this serious complication of heparin therapy.

The constant investigation further elucidates the intricacies of HIT pathophysiology and endeavors to enhance patient outcomes via targeted interventions and therapies.

CHAPTER TWO

Types Of Heparin-Induced Thrombocytopenia

1. Class I HIT:

• Heparin induces a non-immune-mediated type I HIT.

It commonly manifests during the initial one to four days of heparin treatment.

• A modest, transient decrease in platelet count, which is frequently not clinically significant, characterizes type I HIT.

2. Class II HIT:

• Type II HIT is the most severe as it is an immune-mediated reaction.

• It typically develops 5–14 days after heparin exposure; however, re-exposure may accelerate the onset.

Type II HIT is characterized by the generation of IgG antibodies that target the complex formed between heparin and platelet factor 4 (PF4).

• Platelet activation by these antibodies results in thrombocytopenia, platelet consumption, and, ironically, an elevated risk of thrombosis.

Mechanisms Of Development Of HIT

1. Antibody Constructing:

• Heparin forms a complex with PF4, a protein that is liberated from activated platelets.

• PF4 undergoes a conformational change induced by this complex, rendering it immunogenic.

IgG antibodies are generated in response to the heparin-PF4 complex, resulting in platelet activation mediated by the immune system.

2. Platelet stimulation involves:

• Platelet activation is induced when IgG antibodies adhere to the heparin-PF4 complex on platelet surfaces.

• Activated platelets, despite thrombocytopenia, contribute to thrombosis by releasing prothrombotic factors.

3. The Production of Thrombin:

• Thrombin production is stimulated by platelet activation and aggregation, resulting in a hypercoagulable state.

• Due to thrombin's pivotal function in thrombus formation, the risk of arterial and venous thrombosis is increased.

4. Impaired Endothelial Function:

• HIT can result in the activation and dysfunction of endothelial cells, which promotes thrombosis further.

• The aforementioned dysfunction plays a role in the pathophysiology of thrombotic complications observed in HIT.

Manifestations Of HIT In The Clinic

1. Thrombocytopenia is characterized by:

• The platelet count generally declines to below $150 \times 10^9/L$, or less than 50% of its initial value.

• Thrombocytopenia typically develops 5–14 days following heparin exposure; however, re-exposure may accelerate the process.

Mild hemorrhage or petechiae may manifest as a result of a reduced platelet count.

2. Thrombosis occurs when:

• HIT is associated with an elevated risk of arterial and venous thrombosis, notwithstanding thrombocytopenia.

Venous thrombosis frequently impacts deep vessels, which can result in the development of deep vein thrombosis (DVT) or pulmonary embolism (PE).

Arterial thrombosis may present itself in the form of myocardial infarction, limb ischemia, or stroke.

3. Dermal Lesions:

• Heparin-induced skin necrosis (HISN), which occurs at the sites of heparin administration, is a potential adverse effect, particularly when unfractionated heparin is utilized.

4. The dysfunction of organs:

• Vital organ thrombosis may result in failure or dysfunction, including renal or hepatic impairment.

Multiorgan thrombosis has the potential to give rise to severe complications, such as disseminated intravascular coagulation (DIC).

5. Systems for Healthcare Scoring:

• Various scoring systems, including the 4Ts score, are employed to evaluate the pre-test probability of HIT by clinical characteristics.

• Management decisions and diagnostic evaluations are guided by these scores.

In brief, HIT is an intricate immune-mediated response to heparin therapy that is distinguished by thrombocytopenia and an elevated propensity for thrombosis. It is imperative to comprehend the various types, mechanisms, and clinical presentations of this condition to promptly identify it and implement suitable treatment to avert potentially fatal complications.

HIT Laboratory Testing And Diagnosis

Critical diagnosis of HIT is required due to the life-threatening complications that can develop, including arterial and venous thrombosis. The diagnosis is established upon the support of laboratory testing and clinical suspicion. A variety of diagnostic instruments are at one's disposal, encompassing functional assays, clinical scoring systems, and immunoassays.

1. Clinical Evaluation: Clinical evaluation is a crucial component in the diagnosis of HIT. At heparin injection sites, physicians should be on the lookout for signs and symptoms including an abrupt decline in platelet count (typically greater

than 50% from baseline), new or worsening thrombosis, and skin changes.

2. Scoring Systems: To determine the likelihood of HIT, the 4T score is a widely utilized clinical scoring system. It evaluates the severity, chronology, presence of thrombocytopenia, indications of thrombosis, and potential alternative causes of thrombocytopenia. Greater scores correspond to an increased probability of HIT.

3. Immunoassays identify antibodies that target platelet factor 4 (PF4)/heparin complexes, which play a pivotal role in the pathophysiological mechanisms underlying HIT. Particle gel immunoassays (PaGIA) and enzyme-linked immunosorbent assays (ELISA) are both frequently employed immunoassay techniques. It is critical to emphasize, nevertheless, that a positive immunoassay result does not definitively establish the diagnosis of HIT; in fact, antibodies may be present in up to

50% of patients who do not exhibit clinical manifestations of HIT.

4. Functional assays evaluate the capacity of serum from a patient to stimulate platelet activation when heparin is present. Functional assays include the serotonin release assay (SRA) and the heparin-induced platelet activation (HIPA) assay. Although these tests provide a more precise diagnosis of HIT, they might not be universally accessible in all clinical environments.

CHAPTER THREE

Diagnosis Differential For HIT

To prevent misdiagnosis and avoidable treatment cessation, it is critical to conduct a differential diagnosis as numerous conditions may exhibit clinical manifestations similar to HIT. The following conditions ought to be incorporated into the differential diagnosis of HIT:

1.   Additional   Factors   Influencing Thrombocytopenia: In   addition   to   HIT, disseminated   intravascular   coagulation   (DIC), immune   thrombocytopenic   purpura   (ITP),   and drug-induced thrombocytopenia can all contribute to thrombocytopenia.

2. Venous thromboembolism (VTE): Although thrombosis is characteristic of deep vein thrombosis (HIT), it can also manifest in a range of other conditions, such as pulmonary embolism

(PE) and deep vein thrombosis (DVT), which warrant exclusion.

3. Antiphospholipid Syndrome (APS): In the presence of antiphospholipid antibodies, APS is characterized by thrombosis and/or pregnancy complications. The clinical characteristics of APS and HIT may overlap, requiring meticulous evaluation.

4. Disseminated intravascular coagulation (DIC) is a multifaceted condition distinguished by the systemic induction of coagulation, which may result in thrombosis and thrombocytopenia. It can be difficult to distinguish clinically from HIT.

Factors Contributing To The Development Of HIT

Although HIT can occur in any patient undergoing heparin therapy, the risk is increased by the following:

1. Exposure to Heparin for an Extended period: Extended heparin exposure elevates the likelihood of developing HIT. Individuals whose heparin exposure duration exceeds four days are at greater risk in comparison to those whose exposure durations are shorter.

2. HIT is a potential complication of low molecular weight heparin (LMWH) and unfractionated heparin (UFH); however, the likelihood of HIT developing is potentially greater with UFH.

3. Surgery and Intensive Care: The extended administration of heparin for thromboprophylaxis poses an elevated risk to patients undergoing significant surgical procedures, especially those involving the cardiovascular and orthopedic systems. Additionally, the risk is increased for critically ill patients in intensive care units who are administered heparin for thromboprophylaxis.

4. Prior Heparin Exposure: Individuals who have had prior heparin exposure, particularly if they developed hepatotoxicity-induced thrombocytopenia (HIT), are at a heightened risk of experiencing a recurrence of the condition.

5. Patients who have specific underlying conditions, including cancer, autoimmune diseases, and cardiovascular disorders, may have an increased susceptibility to HIT.

6. Advanced age and female gender have been recognized as prospective risk factors for HIT; however, the precise mechanisms that contribute to these correlations remain incompletely elucidated.

Clinicians can identify patients who are more susceptible to developing HIT and implement appropriate preventative and monitoring measures by gaining an understanding of these risk factors. Prompt identification and intervention are critical in mitigating the potential for thrombotic complications linked to HIT.

Complications That Are Linked To HIT

1. Thrombosis is the most severe complication of HIT; if not promptly treated, it can result in substantial morbidity and mortality. Thrombotic events have the potential to impact both the venous and arterial systems, necessitating the implementation of stringent anticoagulation therapy.

2. Organ Ischemia: Ischemia of the limbs, bowel, or myocardium, as well as ischemic stroke and myocardial infarction, may result from thrombosis associated with HIT. Urgent intervention is necessary to prevent tissue injury or organ failure in the face of these complications.

3. Disseminated Intravascular Coagulation (DIC): Life-threatening DIC is distinguished by extensive

microvascular thrombosis and the depletion of clotting factors and platelets. It can result from the widespread activation of the coagulation cascade in severe cases of HIT.

4. Bleeding Associated with Thrombocytopenia: Inexplicably, although thrombocytopenia is a defining characteristic of HIT, it does not occur frequently as a complication. Nevertheless, patients might encounter hemorrhage in certain circumstances as a result of underlying coagulopathy or invasive procedures. Constant vigilance is required to control these possible hemorrhage complications.

Strategies For The Management And Treatment Of HIT

1. Prompt Elimination of Heparin: Discontinuing all formulations of heparin, including unfractionated heparin (UFH) and low molecular weight heparin (LMWH), is the initial course of

action in the management of HIT. Preventing additional platelet activation and thrombus formation is of the utmost importance.

2. Alternative Anticoagulation: To prevent thrombosis while avoiding heparin exposure, patients with HIT require alternative anticoagulation. In addition to fondaparinux, alternatives consist of direct thrombin inhibitors (DTIs) including argatroban, bivalirudin, and lepirudin.

3. Platelet transfusion is typically refrained from in HIT unless patients are experiencing active hemorrhage or necessitate immediate surgical intervention. Platelets that have been transfused may undergo activation when anti-PF4/heparin antibodies are present, thereby worsening thrombosis.

4. It is critical to closely monitor platelet counts and clinical status to detect and assess potential

complications such as hemorrhage or thrombosis. Generally, platelet counts begin to increase again a few days following heparin discontinuation.

5. Anticoagulation Duration: The length of time anticoagulation is administered in patients with HIT is determined by patient-specific factors and the presence of thrombosis. To prevent recurrence, anticoagulation is typically maintained for several months in patients with thrombosis associated with HIT.

CHAPTER FOUR

Pharmaceutical Treatments For HIT

1. Direct Thrombin Inhibitors (DTIs): Because of their capacity to inhibit thrombin directly, DTIs are the agents of choice for anticoagulation in HIT, eliminating the necessity for heparin. Common DTIs include argatroban, bivalirudin, and lepirudin, all of which have distinct pharmacokinetic profiles.

2. Fondaparinux, a synthetic pentasaccharide, selectively inhibits factor Xa, rendering it a compelling substitute for the management of HIT. In contrast to DTIs, their effectiveness in HIT-associated thrombosis is less well-established.

3. Warfarin is typically withheld from administration during the acute phase of HIT on account of its potential for paradoxical thrombosis and delayed onset of action in the presence of

transient protein C depletion. After the patient's platelet counts have stabilized and they are no longer requiring alternative anticoagulants, warfarin may be contemplated as a long-term anticoagulant, often in conjunction with overlapping DTI therapy.

4. Alternative Agents: Further research has been conducted on alternative agents, including danaparoid and direct oral anticoagulants (DOACs), to manage HIT. However, their efficacy is still uncertain and their application may be restricted to particular clinical situations or contraindications to other agents.

HIT is, in summary, a significant adverse effect of heparin therapy that is distinguished by immune-mediated thrombocytopenia and an elevated risk of thrombosis. The timely identification and suitable treatment of complications that have the potential to be fatal are of utmost importance. Proficient approaches to management encompass the prompt discontinuation of heparin, substitution of fondaparinux or DTIs for anticoagulation, and vigilant observation to identify any complications involving thrombosis or hemorrhage.

Non-Pharmaceutical Strategies For The Management Of Hits

1. Irrespective of the cause, the principal non-pharmacological strategy for managing HIT entails discontinuing all heparin products promptly, such as low-molecular-weight heparin (LMWH) and unfractionated heparin. Preventing additional platelet activation and thrombus formation is of the utmost importance.

2. Alternative Anticoagulation: It is imperative to promptly initiate alternative anticoagulants that do not undergo cross-reactivity with HIT antibodies upon diagnosis or suspicion of HIT. Direct thrombin inhibitors (DTIs), including argatroban, bivalirudin, and danaparoid, are among the

available options. Without requiring cofactors such as antithrombin III, these agents inhibit thrombin directly, rendering them efficacious in HIT.

3. It is critical to closely monitor platelet counts and indicators of thrombosis throughout the management of HIT. It is advisable to conduct platelet count monitoring daily or more frequently, particularly in the early stages of treatment.

4. The effective management of thrombosis in patients with HIT is of the utmost importance and requires the use of anticoagulation therapy. Therapeutic doses of DTIs or other non-heparin anticoagulants may be required, depending on the clinical condition of the patient.

5. Surgical Considerations: It is critical to exercise meticulous risk management of thrombosis and effectively coordinate anticoagulation in HIT patients who necessitate surgery.

A multidisciplinary approach comprising surgeons, anesthesiologists, and hematologists is advised, in addition to consultation with a hematologist.

Long-Term Prognosis And Results Of HIT

The prognosis for HIT is predominantly influenced by the timeliness of diagnosis, administration of suitable treatment, and control of thrombotic complications. Type I HIT generally resolves without any enduring repercussions, whereas type II HIT is notoriously linked to substantial morbidity and mortality as a result of thrombotic complications.

In the absence of proper management, deep vein thrombosis (HIT) can result in severe thrombotic complications, including pulmonary embolism (PE), stroke, myocardial infarction (MI), limb ischemia, and potentially fatal outcomes.

Thrombosis is an especially prevalent complication among individuals who have type II HIT.

Several factors, including the severity of thrombotic complications, the presence of comorbidities, and the patient's response to anticoagulation therapy, influence the long-term outcomes of HIT. Despite adequate treatment, certain patients may develop chronic complications, such as post-thrombotic syndrome or recurrent thrombosis.

CHAPTER FIVE

Patient Support And Education Regarding HIT

To ensure early detection of symptoms, prevention of complications, and adherence to therapy, patient education and support are vital elements of HIT management. Critical elements of patient education and support comprise:

1. Comprehending HIT: Disseminating thorough information to patients regarding HIT, encompassing its etiology, manifestations, potential complications, and therapeutic alternatives.

2. Plaque count monitoring and adherence to alternative anticoagulation therapy should be emphasized as critical components of medication management.

3. Symptom Identification: Informing patients regarding the indications and manifestations of thrombosis, including extremity edema, pain, erythema, angina, dyspnea, and neurological impairments.

4. Lifestyle Modifications: Suggest to patients that they adopt lifestyle modifications, such as maintaining a healthy weight, engaging in regular exercise, quitting smoking, and avoiding protracted immobility, to mitigate the risk of thrombosis.

5. Facilitating the connection between patients and HIT support groups or online communities provides an avenue for the exchange of personal anecdotes, emotional solace, and access to beneficial resources.

6. Subsequent Care: Consistently maintain follow-up appointments with healthcare providers to monitor progress, make necessary adjustments to

therapy, and address any complications that may arise.

Guidelines And Prevention Strategies For HIT

The mitigation of HIT is contingent upon the reduction of heparin usage and the implementation of suitable approaches for identifying and managing patients who are at risk. Crucial preventive measures and recommendations encompass:

1. Risk Assessment: Perform an exhaustive risk assessment to identify patients who are at an elevated risk of developing thrombotic thrombocytopenia (HIT), such as those with a prior HIT diagnosis, recent heparin exposure, or specific medical conditions that promote thrombosis.

2. Alternative Anticoagulants: In patients at high risk for HIT or with a history of HIT, alternative

anticoagulants such as fondaparinux or direct thrombin inhibitors should be considered.

3. Heparin monitoring involves closely observing heparin therapy and discontinuing it promptly in patients who exhibit clinical suspicion of thrombotic events or thrombocytopenia without an explanation.

4. Educational Programs: Encouraging healthcare providers to participate in educational programs that aim to enhance their understanding of HIT, its associated risks, and suitable management approaches.

5. Developing institutional protocols and guidelines for the management of HIT, including algorithms for the prevention, treatment, and diagnosis of thrombosis associated with HIT.

6. Research and Surveillance: Facilitating investigations into the pathophysiology of HIT,

identifying innovative biomarkers, and formulating enhanced therapeutic and diagnostic approaches. In addition, the implementation of surveillance systems to track the occurrence and results of HITs to inform preventative measures.

By amalgamating these methodologies, medical practitioners can efficiently oversee health information technology, reduce complexities, and enhance patient results.

Summary

In summary, Heparin-Induced Thrombocytopenia (HIT) signifies an intricate and conceivably fatal immune-mediated response to the administration of heparin. Clinicians must have a thorough understanding of HIT due to the high rates of morbidity and mortality that can result if it is not promptly identified and managed. As this investigation progresses, it becomes apparent that HIT is distinguished by a paradoxical thrombotic condition in which thrombocytopenia is present, thereby presenting diagnostic difficulties.

Incorporating laboratory tests, clinical assessments, and HIT-specific assays into diagnostic algorithms facilitates risk stratification and timely diagnosis. It is critical to initiate alternative anticoagulation strategies, such as direct thrombin inhibitors, without delay to protect HIT patients from thromboembolic complications.

In addition, HIT emphasizes the significance of interdisciplinary cooperation among healthcare professionals to guarantee timely identification, suitable treatment, and prevention of unfavorable consequences. It is critical to educate patients about the risk factors and symptoms of HIT to facilitate timely detection and intervention.

Further investigation is required to clarify the pathogenesis of HIT, enhance diagnostic methods, and create anticoagulant alternatives that are safer. The cultivation of a holistic comprehension of HIT by healthcare practitioners can enhance patient outcomes and alleviate the potentially catastrophic ramifications linked to this state.

THE END